KARIN KALTEREN BUSINK

The Power of Food Choices

Simple Steps to Transform Your Health and Protect the Earth

This book was professionally typeset on Reedsy.
Find out more at reedsy.com

Contents

1

Introduction

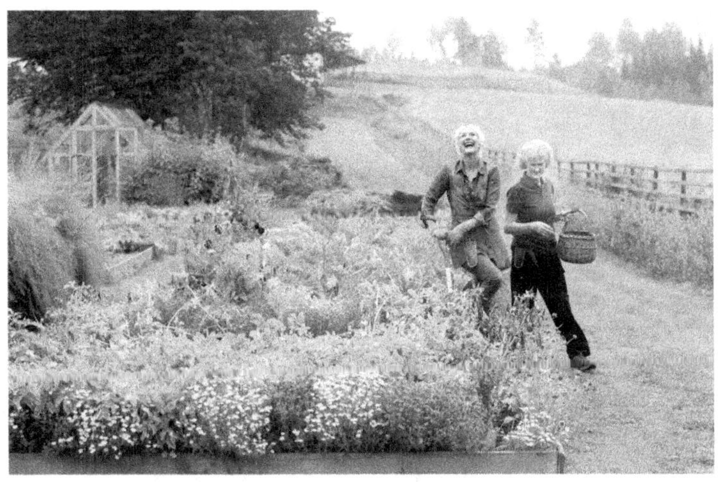

Change your Food, Change the World!

All great things start with one small step, one choice, one decision that moves you forward. Remember the power of the 3C's: Choices, Chances, Changes. You must make a choice to take a chance or your life will never change. It will all lead to my favourite C Celebrate! If you want to eat healthier and want to make better food choices this book is for you.

Many years ago we could not even image what effect AI would have on our society, perhaps many of you still cannot grasp the enormous changes we will encounter in the next 10 years!

But whatever AI will bring, one topic will not change. What unites all of us, regardless of where we live on this planet, is food. Recipes from all corners of the world inspire us to prepare beautiful, complex, and sometimes very simple meals.

However, now we know that the global food chain is currently in a state of serious disruption, causing significant damage to soil and water. It is under immense pressure due to climate change, wars, economic interests, and political unwillingness or, at times, incompetence.

We live in a Food Advertisers World, they are experts at playing on our emotions and convenience. Commercials featuring happy, fit families enjoying a quick meal from a microwave or a snack on the go tap into our desires for both health and ease. These ads suggest that by choosing their product, we can save time and still nourish our bodies. Some claims are even ridiculous and far from healthy at all. The reality is that many of these prepackaged foods are laden with unhealthy fats, excessive sodium, and artificial additives that contribute to long-term health issues like obesity, heart disease, and diabetes.

Misleading advertising has a powerful impact on the food

choices we make, often steering us toward unhealthy pre-packaged options under the guise of convenience and health. By becoming more aware of these tactics and making more informed decisions, we can not only improve our own well-being but also contribute to a healthier, more sustainable world.

The Earth does not cater to us—except to remind us that humanity cannot survive without a healthy planet.

This little smart book is an invitation to rethink your relationship with food. The origin, treatment, and processing of food can make a world of difference for the health and well-being of people, animals, and the environment. I would like to invite you to buy at your Local Farmers market or buy Organic food. All sorts of Diets are fine with me, as long as it's organic. Grass fed beef, or lam . Even if you eat Plant Based, buy organic-Free of pesticides and hormones. Which is good for your health and the planet. So a win-win situation.

The photos in this book are from my organic farm, aiming to inspire you to recognize the importance of organic farming for a healthier life and environment. But they also offer you delicious and simple seasonal recipes.

As a farmer on an organic farm, it's clear to us every day that your perspective on food dramatically changes when you connect with the animals and vegetables you grow.

I will share with you a season on my Organic Farm in the heart of Sweden.

We start in the spring, with the promise of new life and sowing in the garden. We grow lots of vegetables and berries of all sorts. We make our own lemonade and the Apples are pressed at a local farmer to juice. There are lots of vegetables to choose from and we enjoy them throughout the winter. We have big freezers and also ferment vegetables. But if you are not living on a farm, or are not in a position to do it by yourself, then your local Farmers Markets are a perfect Choice!

2

The Importance of Real Food, Farmers' Markets, and Hormone-Free, Pesticide-Free Food

I n a world where convenience often trumps quality, the importance of real food—food that is unprocessed and as close to its natural state as possible—cannot be overstated. Real food is the cornerstone of a healthy lifestyle, contributing not only to personal well-being but also to animal welfare and the sustainability of our planet.

<u>Find your nearest Farmers market.</u> In Sweden we have the REKO -ring , local farmers market. Easy to order directly via the REKO- ring Facebook group. The Farmers' Markets are the best way to access Real Food. It's also nice to know who produces food in the area you live. These markets offer a direct link between consumers and local farmers, fostering a sense of community while ensuring that the food you purchase is fresh, seasonal, and often grown using sustainable practices. Unlike produce found in large supermarkets, which may have

traveled thousands of miles and sat in storage for days or even weeks, the fruits, vegetables, and meats at farmers' markets are typically harvested at peak ripeness, preserving their full nutritional value and flavor.

If you buy lots of fresh runner beans for example - you can freeze them and you can enjoy good food even in the winter. When in season vegetables are cheap and if you buy more to freeze for the winter months, it helps your budget and you are better off.

Farmers' markets are also a hub for food free of hormones and pesticides—another critical factor in promoting health. Hormones are often used in industrial farming to speed up the growth of livestock, while pesticides are commonly applied to crops to ward off insects and other pests. While these practices may increase efficiency, they come at a significant cost. Hormone-laden meat has been linked to various health issues, including early puberty in children and an increased risk of certain cancers. Pesticides, too, pose real health risks, such as neurological problems and an increased risk of cancer, especially for those with high levels of exposure.

Choosing food that is free of hormones and pesticides is not just a personal health decision; it's also an ethical one. Animals raised without synthetic hormones tend to have better living conditions, as they are not forced to grow unnaturally quickly. Similarly, farmers who avoid pesticides often adopt more sustainable farming practices, such as crop rotation and natural pest deterrents, which are better for the environment. These methods help maintain soil health, preserve water quality, and reduce the carbon footprint of food production.

Incorporating real food into your diet, especially from farmers' markets, and opting for hormone-free, pesticide-free options, is a powerful way to contribute to your health, support animal welfare, and promote a healthier planet. It's a step towards a more sustainable future, where the food we eat nourishes our bodies, respects the lives of animals, and protects the Earth for future generations.

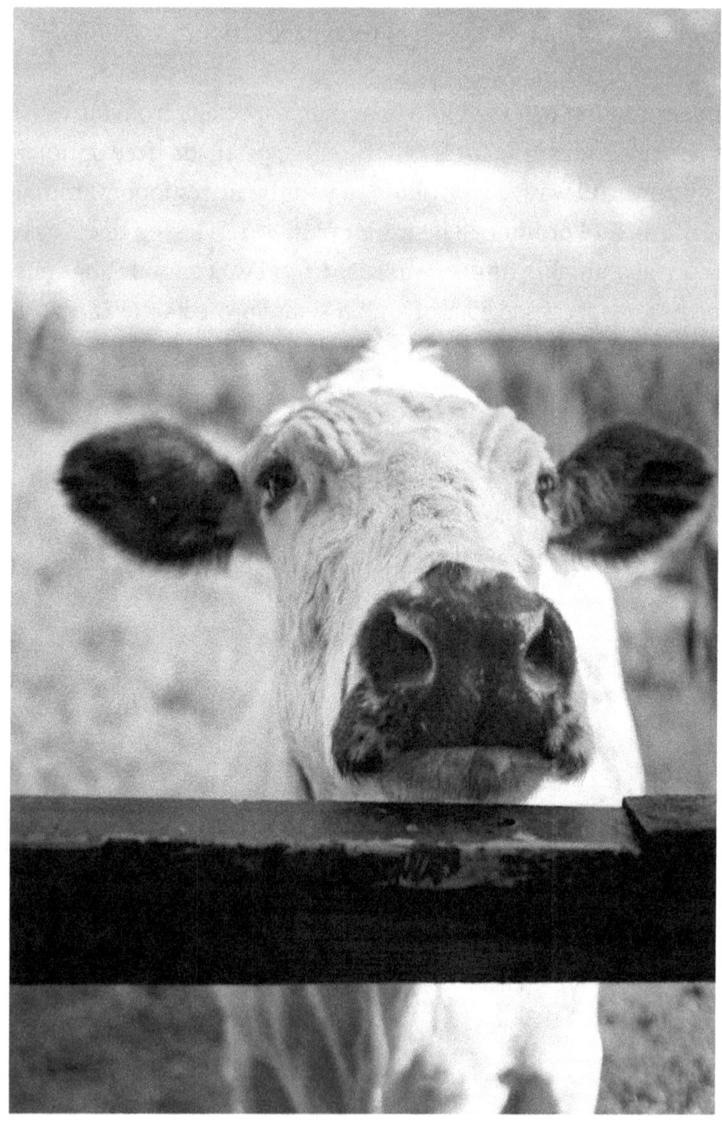

3

Grass-Fed Goodness

I n the quest for healthier living, more people are turning to the source of their food with a greater sense of responsibility and awareness. Among the most impact choices we can make is opting for grass-fed meat and dairy products—a decision that not only benefits our health but also honors the well-being of the animals that sustain us.

Healthy Happy Animal, Healthy Happy You: When animals are raised on a natural diet of grass, the nutritional profile of the meat and dairy they produce is markedly superior to that of their grain-fed counterparts. Grass-fed beef, for example, is richer in essential nutrients like Omega-3 fatty acids, which are known for their anti-inflammatory properties and benefits to heart health. These animals also produce meat that is lower in unhealthy fats and higher in vitamins such as Vitamin E and antioxidants like beta-carotene, which contribute to overall well-being and disease prevention.

For dairy, the story is much the same. Grass-fed cows produce milk with higher levels of Conjugated Linoleic Acid (CLA), a fatty acid that has been shown to support weight loss, improve immune function, and even reduce the risk of certain cancers. The purity and richness of these nutrients reflect the health of the animals themselves—healthy animals naturally yield healthier products.

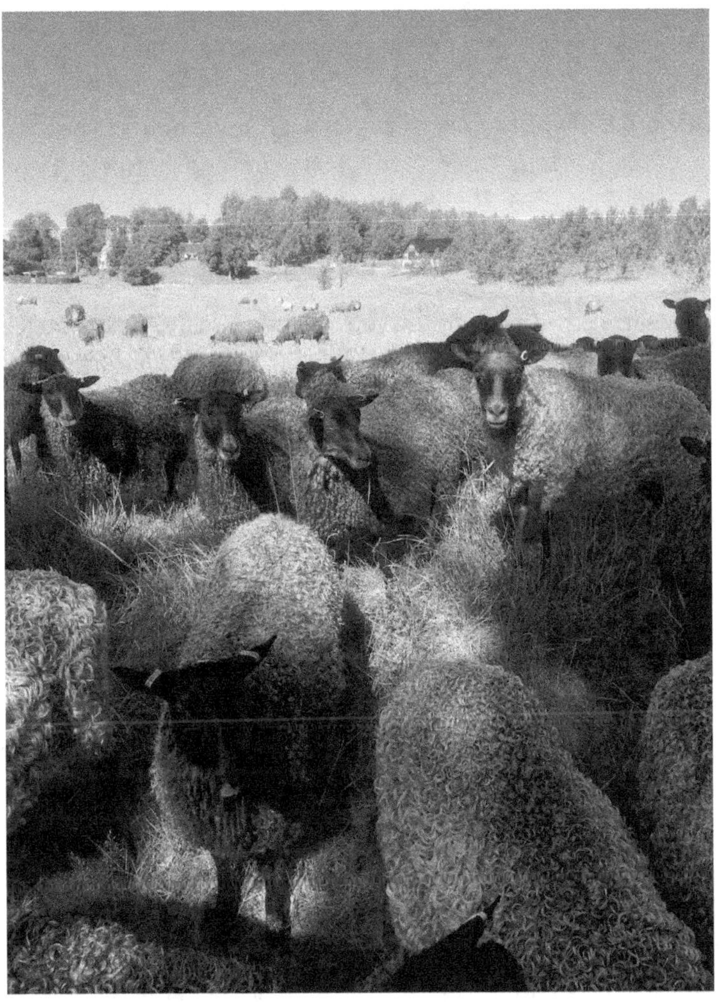

Our Gotland Sheep enjoying the pastures

A Commitment to Animal Welfare

Choosing grass-fed is not just about what's on our plates; it's about how we treat the creatures that provide for us. Animals that are allowed to graze on open pastures lead lives that are more aligned with their natural behaviors and instincts. They roam freely, graze at their own pace, and are not subjected to the cramped, stressful conditions of industrial feedlots.

This humane treatment translates directly into the quality of the food they produce. Animals that live stress-free lives are less likely to require antibiotics and other medications, resulting in cleaner, safer food for us. Moreover, the ethical implications of consuming products from well-treated animals resonate deeply within us, nourishing not just our bodies but also our consciences.

In Harmony with Nature

Grass-fed farming also fosters a harmonious relationship with the environment. Pasture-raised animals contribute to the health of the land, enriching the soil with their manure and promoting biodiversity by grazing on a variety of plants. This regenerative approach to farming stands in stark contrast to the environmental degradation caused by conventional, industrial livestock operations, which are often associated with deforestation, water pollution, and high greenhouse gas emissions.

By choosing grass-fed products, we support farming practices that work in tandem with nature rather than against it. This not only sustains the planet but also ensures that future generations will have access to the same high-quality, nourishing foods.

A Holistic Approach to Health

The benefits of grass-fed animals extend beyond the physical. When we consume food that is wholesome, ethically produced, and environmentally sustainable, we are taking a holistic approach to our health. We acknowledge that what we eat is not just about fueling our bodies—it's about the impact we have on the world around us.

Eating grass-fed meat and dairy is a way of saying yes to a food system that values quality over quantity, health over convenience, and respect over exploitation. It is a powerful reminder that the well-being of the animals we consume cannot be separated from our own.

Grass-fed animals offer us more than just nutrient-rich food; they offer us a way to reconnect with the land, respect the creatures that sustain us, and make choices that reflect our values. By choosing grass-fed products, we nourish our bodies with the best that nature has to offer, while also honouring the lives of the animals that contribute to our health. In this way, we create a cycle of care and respect that ultimately benefits everyone—humans, animals, and the planet alike.

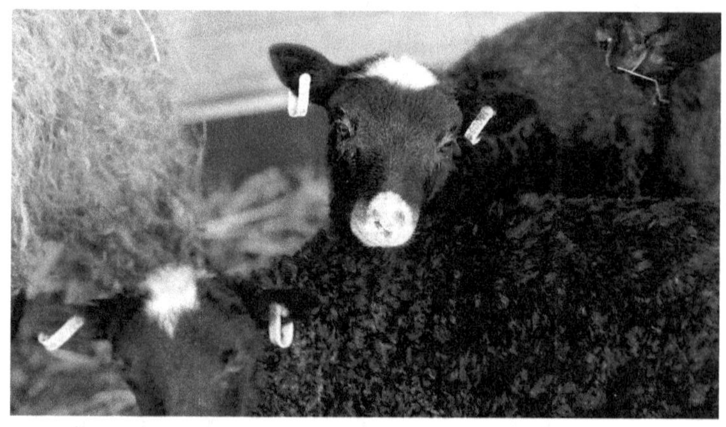

4

A Year on the Farm: Growing with the Moon, Harvesting with Joy

Nestled in the heart of the Swedish Countryside of Värmland, our organic sheep farm and vegetable garden are more than just a way of life—they're a celebration of nature's rhythms and the simple joys of working the land. Here, we've embraced the wisdom of old traditions, the excitement of new beginnings, and the magic that comes from watching seeds grow into bountiful harvests.

Gardening with the Moon

At the core of our farming practices is a deep respect for nature's cycles, and nowhere is this more evident than in our approach to gardening. We follow the ancient practice of gardening with the moon, a method that aligns our planting and harvesting with the lunar phases. This tradition, passed down through generations, teaches us that the moon's gravitational pull influences not only the tides but also the moisture in the soil, encouraging seeds to sprout and plants to thrive.

Each month, as the moon waxes and wanes, we plan our gardening tasks accordingly. The waxing moon, growing fuller each night, is the perfect time to sow seeds that produce above-ground crops—like tomatoes, beans, and leafy greens. As the moon wanes, shrinking back to a slender crescent, we turn our attention to root crops like carrots and potatoes, trusting that this natural rhythm will lead to stronger, more vibrant plants.

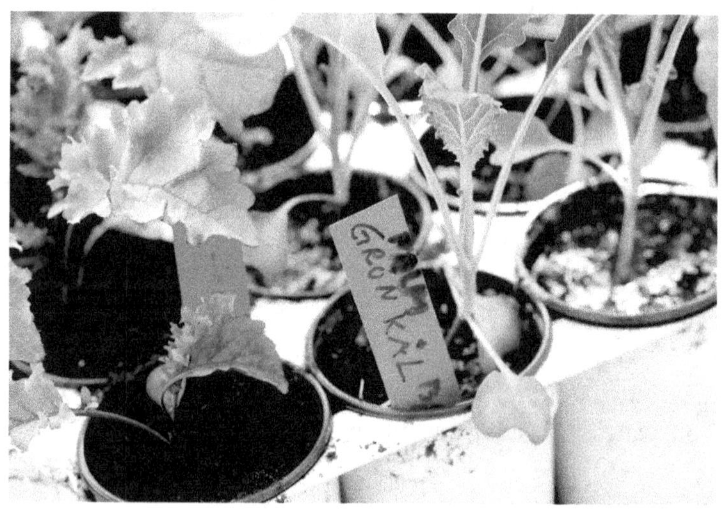

Sowing in the Spring

Spring is a season of hope and renewal on the farm. As the earth warms under the gentle kiss of the sun, we eagerly gather our seeds, ready to start a new cycle of growth. This year, we've chosen to source our seeds from The Bolster, a renowned organic seed company in Holland. Known for their high-quality, sustainably produced seeds, The Bolster offers us the best start possible for our garden. Each packet we open is a promise—a tiny miracle waiting to unfold.

With seeds in hand, we head out to the garden, the soil rich and dark beneath our feet. There's something magical about those first days of spring planting. The air is filled with the scent of freshly turned earth, and the garden buzzes with the quiet energy of new beginnings. As we press each seed into the soil, we can't help but imagine the harvests to come—rows of juicy tomatoes, baskets overflowing with beans, and leafy greens as far as the eye can see.

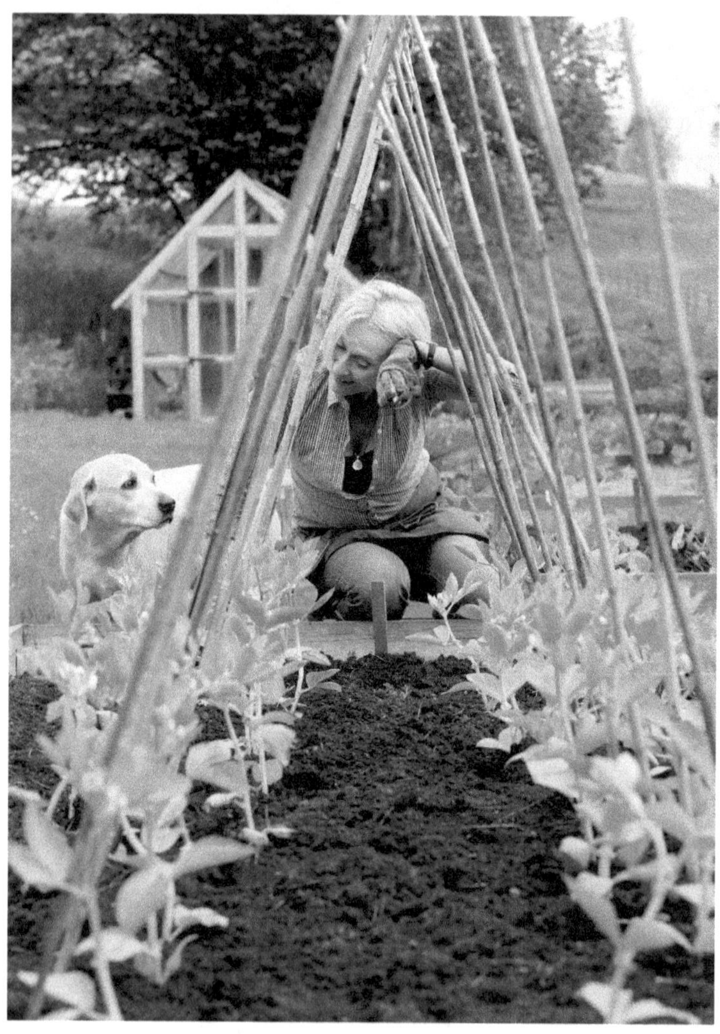

The Joy of Planting

Planting is a joyful, communal experience on our farm. We gather together, friends and family, each taking part in the process. Laughter and conversation flow as easily as the seeds from our hands. There's no rush—just the steady, satisfying rhythm of planting, watering, and nurturing. Each seed we sow is a connection to the land, to each other, and to the future harvest.

As we work, we imagine how the garden will look in the height of summer, when the plants have grown tall and strong. We talk about the meals we'll prepare, the flavours we'll savor, and the satisfaction of knowing that we grew it all ourselves. There's a sense of anticipation in the air—a feeling that we're part of something much bigger than ourselves.

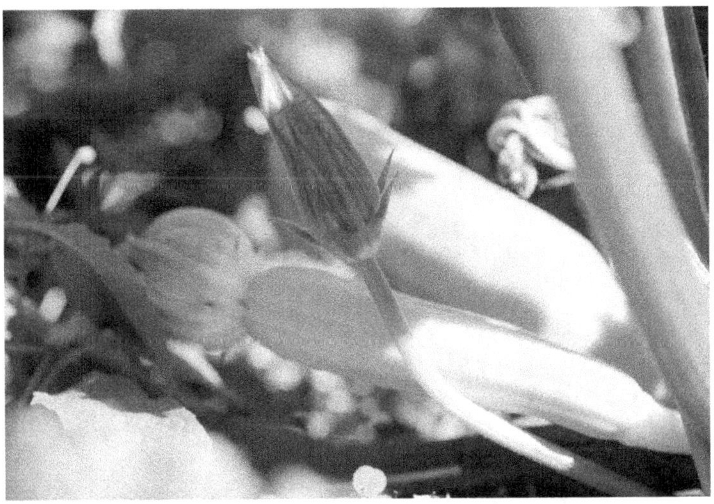

Harvesting with Gratitude

As the seasons change, our garden transforms before our eyes.

The seeds we planted in spring have grown into a lush, abundant garden, filled with vibrant colors and rich aromas. Harvest time is the reward for all our hard work, and it's every bit as joyful as we imagined.

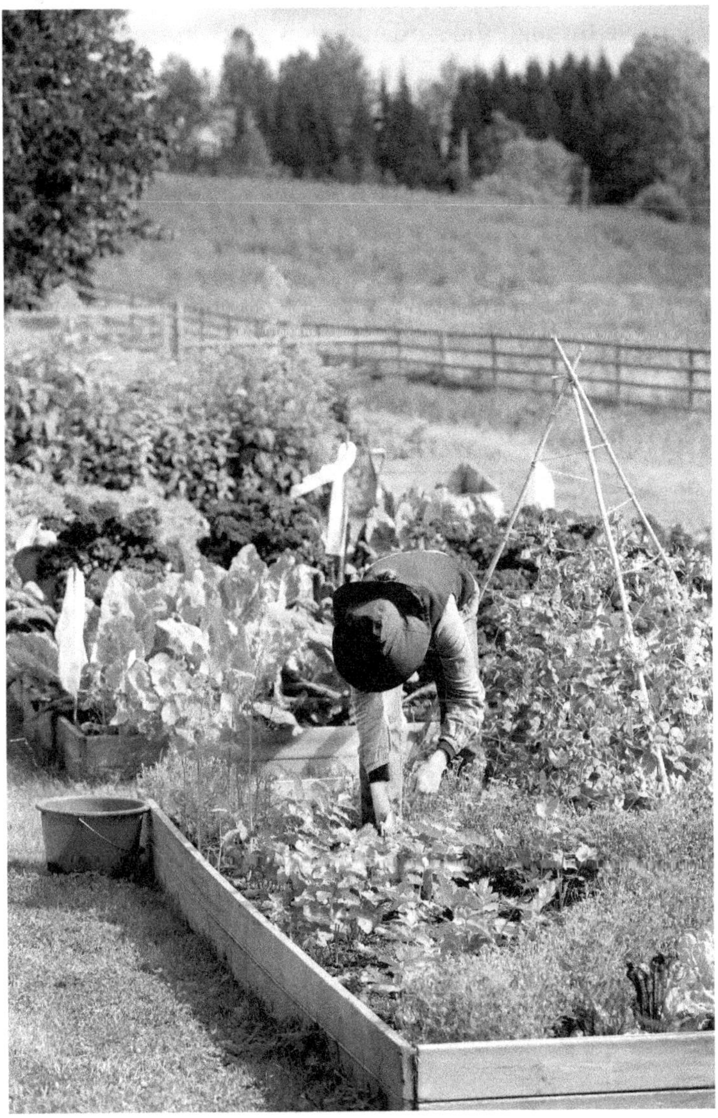

We move through the garden with baskets in hand, picking tomatoes that are warm from the sun, pulling carrots from the earth, and gathering greens for our evening meal. The sheep graze contentedly in the nearby pasture, their woolly coats soft against the backdrop of a golden autumn sunset. There's a deep sense of gratitude that fills us as we harvest—a recognition that we're not just taking from the earth, but participating in a cycle of giving and receiving.

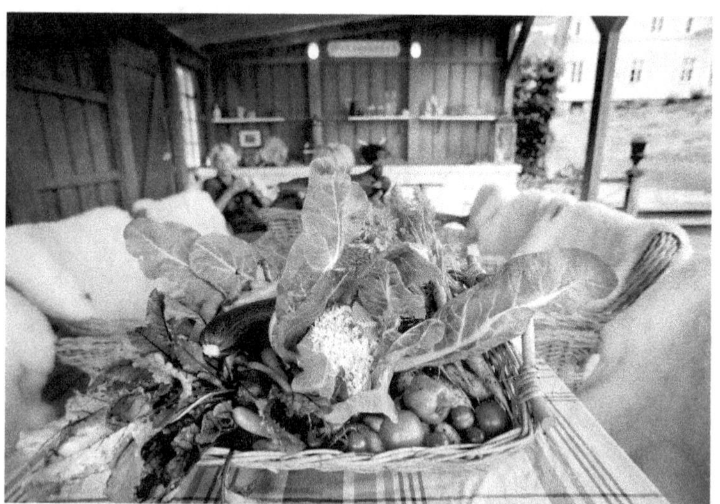

5

Choose Your Greens Wisely: The Hidden Truth About Prepackaged and Sprayed Produce.

It's easy to reach for prepackaged vegetables or shiny apples that seem to promise freshness and ease. But beneath the surface, these seemingly simple choices can have hidden consequences for both our health and the environment. It's time to take a closer look at what we're putting on our plates and learn how to choose our greens wisely. Freeze homemade tomato sauce! Buy your tomato's at the Farmers markets. You be surprised to find different sorts than in the supermarket, and much more taste!

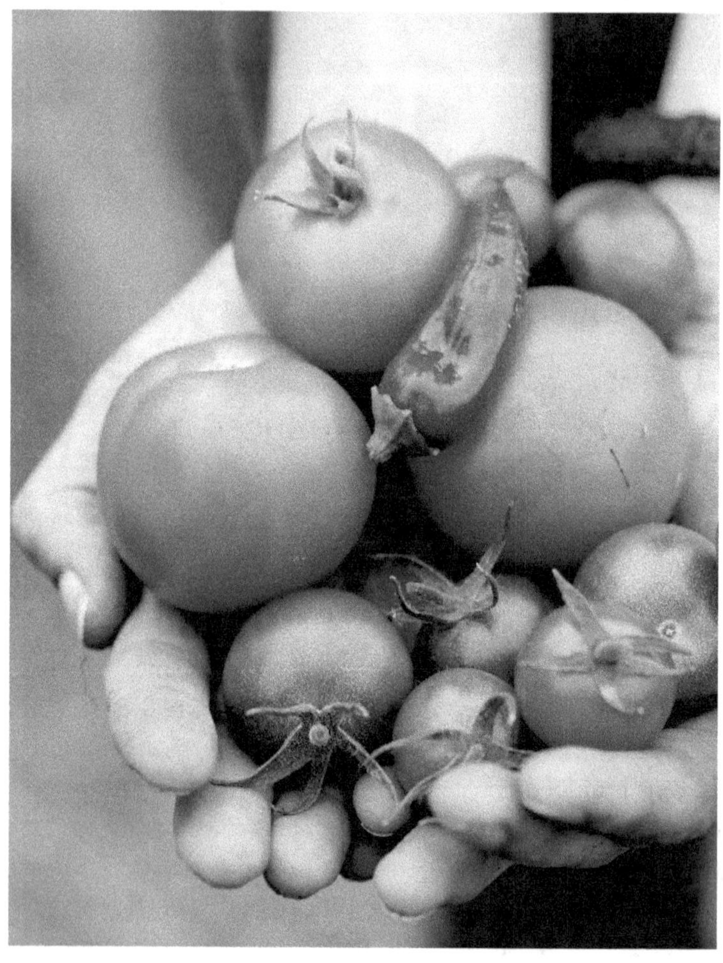

The Hidden Dangers of Prepackaged Vegetables

Prepackaged vegetables may seem like a quick and healthy option, but many of these products come with a catch. To keep the produce looking fresh and to extend its shelf life, companies often seal these vegetables in packaging filled with gases like carbon dioxide or nitrogen. While these gases are not harmful in themselves, the process can strip the vegetables of some of their nutrients and flavor. Moreover, the plastic packaging contributes to environmental pollution, adding to the already overwhelming problem of plastic waste.

Another concern is the loss of freshness. Once vegetables are cut, they begin to lose nutrients more rapidly, and prepackaged vegetables, which are often pre-cut, can be significantly less nutritious than their whole, unpackaged counterparts.

By the time they reach your plate, they may have lost much of their vitality.

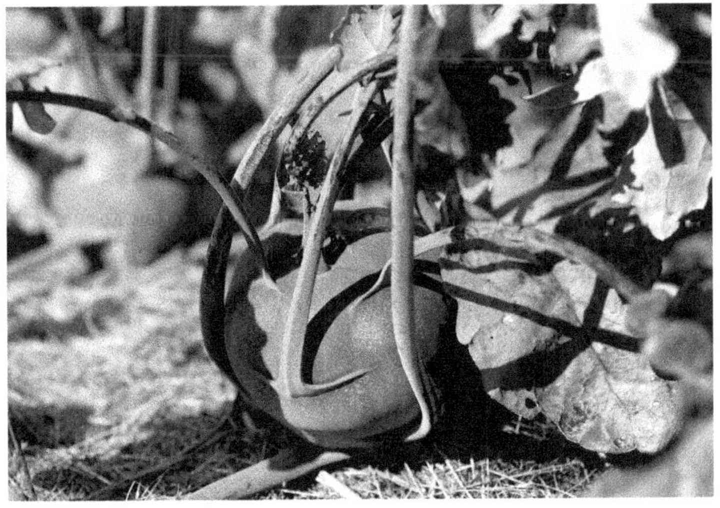

6

The Reality of Sprayed Produce

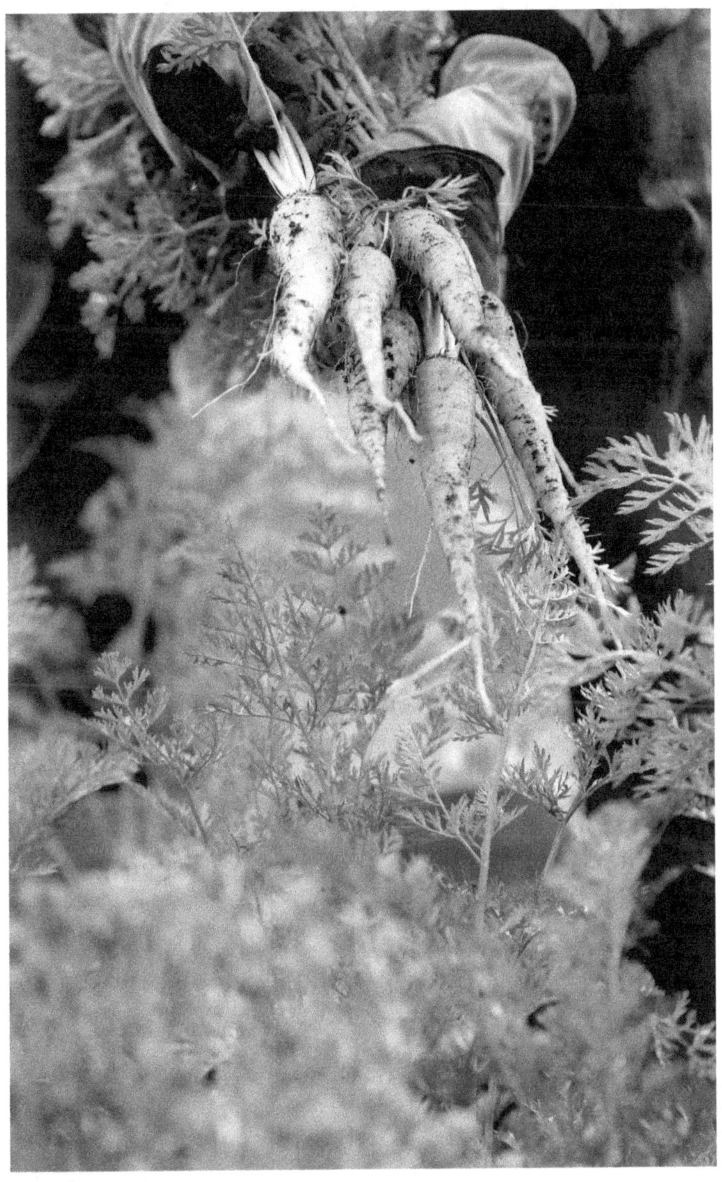

Change to Making Better Choices: Go Organic and Local

To protect your health and the environment, consider these tips when choosing your produce:

1. Buy Organic: Whenever possible, choose organic fruits and vegetables. Organic farming practices avoid the use of synthetic pesticides and fertilizers, reducing your exposure to harmful chemicals. Organic produce is also more likely to be fresher, as it's often sold locally and in season.

2. Visit Farmers' Markets: Local farmers' markets are a treasure trove of fresh, seasonal produce. Here, you can talk directly to the growers, learn about their farming practices, and often find organic or minimally treated fruits and vegetables. Supporting local farmers also helps to reduce the carbon footprint associated with transporting produce over long distances.

3. Wash Thoroughly: If you can't always buy organic, make sure to wash your fruits and vegetables thoroughly. Use a vegetable brush for firm produce and a mixture of water and vinegar to help remove some of the pesticides on softer items. Peeling fruits like apples can also reduce your exposure, though this might remove some nutrients as well.

4. Grow Your Own: If you have the space, consider starting a small garden. Growing your own vegetables ensures that you know exactly what's going into your food. Even a few pots on a balcony can yield fresh herbs, tomatoes, or leafy greens.

5. Choose Whole Foods: Whenever possible, buy whole fruits and vegetables rather than pre-cut or prepackaged options.

6. Whole produce retains its nutrients better and avoids the need for gas-filled packaging.

7

The Perils of Plastic: Protecting Our Oceans and Choosing Seafood Wisely

We are fortunate to live in Sweden with her wonderful lakes and fresh waters! The rivers are clean and our local lake Värmeln holds lovely fish to catch if you like to fish.

Our oceans, once pristine and teeming with life, are now facing an unprecedented threat: plastic pollution. From the smallest plankton to the largest whales, marine life is being affected by the millions of tons of plastic that enter the oceans each year. As consumers, it's crucial to be aware of the impact this has on the seafood we eat and the steps we can take to protect both our health and the environment. First step is to **Recycle Plastic** and trow nothing in nature or the sea. Or even better deposit on plastics.

The Plastic Invasion

Plastic is everywhere—packaging, bottles, bags, and countless other everyday items. Unfortunately, a significant amount of this plastic ends up in the ocean, where it breaks down into tiny particles known as microplastics. These microplastics are now found throughout the marine environment, from the surface waters to the deepest ocean trenches. It should be teached at schools, and at home as well to RECYCLE and not throw plastic in Nature where it does not belong.

Marine animals, including fish, mistake these tiny plastic particles for food. Once ingested, the plastic can cause physical harm, block digestive tracts, and even lead to death. But the problem doesn't end there. When we consume seafood, we're also consuming the microplastics that have accumulated in these animals' bodies.

Microplastics in Seafood: A Hidden Danger

Recent studies have shown that microplastics are present in a wide range of seafood, including fish, shellfish, and even sea salt. While the long-term health effects of consuming microplastics are still being studied, there is growing concern about the potential risks. Microplastics can carry toxic chemicals that may accumulate in our bodies over time, leading to possible health issues.

The presence of microplastics in fish is a stark reminder of the interconnections of our environment and our food supply. What happens in the ocean eventually finds its way onto our plates, highlighting the need for more responsible consumption and greater efforts to reduce plastic pollution.

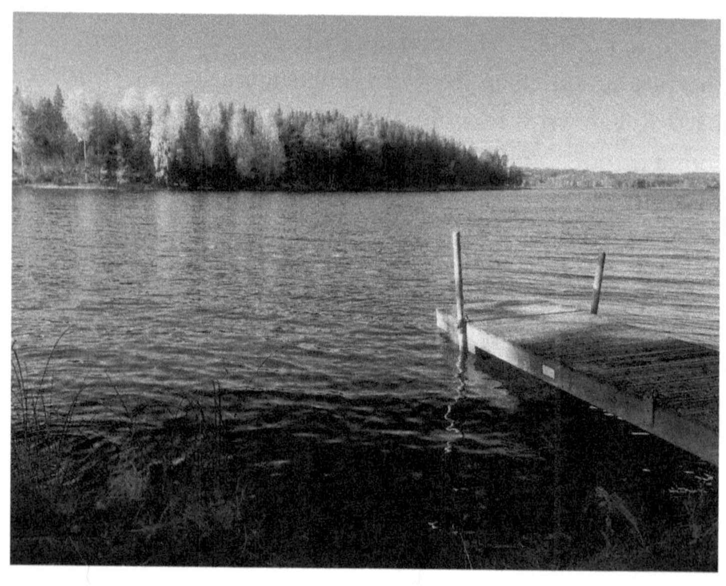

8

Choosing your Seafood Wisely

Given the prevalence of plastic pollution and the challenges it poses, it's more important than ever to be mindful of where and what we buy when it comes to seafood. Here are some tips to help you make safer and more sustainable choices:

1. **Know Your Source:** Be aware of where your seafood comes from. Fish caught in heavily polluted waters are more likely to contain microplastics and other contaminants. When possible, choose seafood from cleaner, less industrialised areas.

2. **Support Sustainable Fishing Practices:** Opt for seafood that is sourced from sustainable fisheries, which often take extra measures to ensure the health of the ocean and the fish populations. Look for certifications like the Marine Stewardship Council (MSC) or Aquaculture Stewardship Council (ASC) when shopping.

3. **Limit Consumption of Certain Fish:** Some fish species,

particularly those lower on the food chain like small, oily fish (e.g., sardines, anchovies), are less likely to accumulate high levels of microplastics compared to larger predatory fish like tuna and swordfish. By choosing smaller fish, you can reduce your exposure to these contaminants.

4. **Consider Freshwater Alternatives:** If you're fortunate enough to have access to clean rivers and lakes, consider fishing there. Freshwater fish, especially from well-maintained, pollution-free areas, are less likely to contain microplastics compared to their ocean-dwelling counterparts. Always ensure that the water source is clean and the fish population is healthy before fishing.

5. **Reduce Plastic Use:** One of the most impactful steps we can take as individuals is to reduce our use of single-use plastics. By cutting down on plastic waste, we can help prevent more plastic from entering the ocean. Simple actions like using reusable bags, bottles, and containers can make a big difference.

6. **Advocate for Change:** Support policies and initiatives aimed at reducing plastic pollution and promoting ocean conservation. Whether it's participating in beach cleanups, advocating for bans on single-use plastics, or supporting organisations that work to protect marine environments, your voice and actions matter.

The ocean's health is intimately connected to our own. As plastic continues to invade our seas, it's crucial that we become more conscious consumers, not just for the sake of the environment but for our own well-being. By making informed choices about the seafood we eat, reducing our plastic use, and supporting sustainable practices, we can help protect the oceans and ensure that future generations can enjoy the bounty of the sea—without the hidden dangers of plastic.

9

Alternatives to Animal Proteins, the New Green Protein.

Pulses and Their Power as Plant-Based Alternatives

As more people embrace healthier and more sustainable lifestyles, the demand for alternatives to animal proteins has grown. Enter pulses—a diverse group of leguminous crops that includes beans, lentils, chickpeas, and peas. These humble yet powerful plants are emerging as key players in the movement toward plant-based diets, offering a wealth of nutritional benefits and culinary versatility. Whether you're looking to reduce your meat consumption, explore new flavors, or simply add more variety to your meals, pulses are a fantastic option.

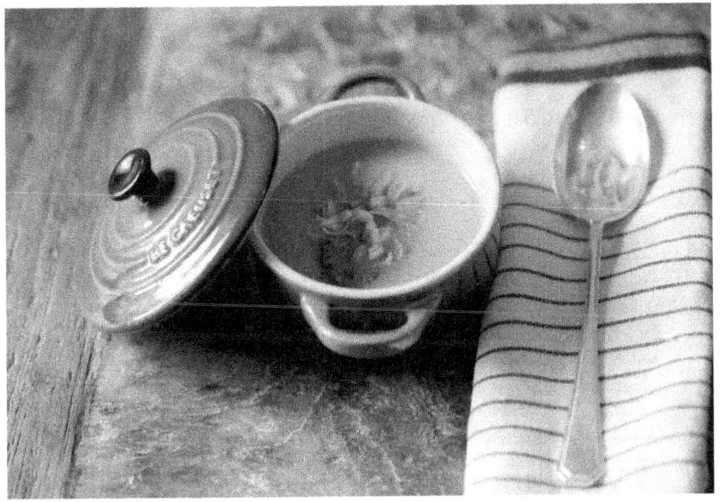

What Are Pulses?

Pulses are a type of legume harvested for their dry seeds. They include:

- Beans: Varieties like black beans, kidney beans, navy beans, and pinto beans.
- Lentils: Available in colours ranging from green and brown to red, yellow, and black.
- Chickpeas (Garbanzo Beans): Popular in Middle Eastern and Mediterranean cuisines.
- Peas: Such as split peas and whole dried peas.

Pulses are not only packed with protein but also rich in fiber, vitamins, and minerals, making them a nutritious and sustainable alternative to animal-based proteins.

Nutritional Benefits of Pulses

Pulses are often referred to as "green proteins" because they are both environmentally friendly and highly nutritious. Here's why they're worth adding to your diet:

1. High Protein Content: Pulses are an excellent source of plant-based protein, essential for building and repairing tissues. For those looking to reduce or eliminate meat, pulses offer a protein-rich alternative that can help meet daily requirements.
2. Rich in Fibres: Pulses are loaded with dietary fibre, which aids digestion, helps regulate blood sugar levels, and supports heart health. The fibre in pulses also promotes a feeling of fullness, making them a great option for weight management.
3. Packed with Micro nutrients: Pulses are rich in essential vitamins and minerals, including iron, folate, magnesium, and potassium. They also contain antioxidants that help protect the body from oxidative stress.
4. Low in Fat: Most pulses are low in fat and contain no cholesterol, making them heart-healthy alternatives to animal proteins.
5. Environmental Sustainability: Growing pulses requires less water and energy compared to animal farming. They also help improve soil health by fixing nitrogen, reducing the need for synthetic fertilisers.

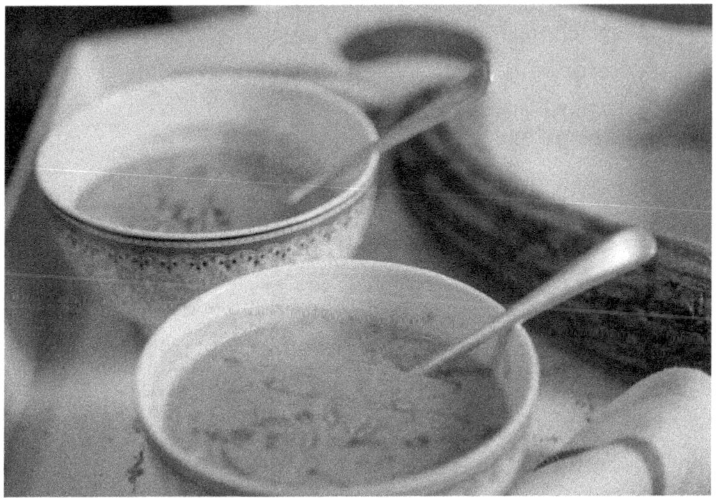

Culinary Versatility: How to Use Pulses in Your Diet

One of the greatest advantages of pulses is their versatility in the kitchen. They can be used in a wide range of dishes, from soups and stews to salads and snacks. Here are some creative ways to incorporate pulses into your meals:

1. Hearty Soups and Stews: Pulses add substance and protein to soups and stews. Lentils, chickpeas, and split peas cook quickly and absorb flavours beautifully. Try a warming lentil soup or a robust chickpea stew for a satisfying meal.
2. Salads with a Protein Punch: Toss cooked beans or lentils into salads to boost their protein content. A black bean and corn salad with avocado, or a Mediterranean chickpea salad with tomatoes, cucumbers, and olives, makes for a delicious and nutritious dish.
3. Plant-Based Burgers: Pulses are the star ingredients in

many plant-based burger recipes. Mash cooked black beans or lentils with spices, oats, and vegetables to create tasty patties that can be grilled or baked.

4. Dips and Spreads: Hummus, made from chickpeas, is a classic example of how pulses can be turned into creamy, flavorful spreads. Experiment with different pulses like white beans or lentils to create your own unique dips.

5. Curries and Stir-Fries: Pulses work wonderfully in curries and stir-fries, absorbing spices and sauces. Try a red lentil curry with coconut milk or a stir-fry with tofu and green peas for a protein-packed meal.

6. Pasta and Grain Bowls: Add cooked lentils, chickpeas, or beans to pasta dishes and grain bowls for extra protein and texture. A lentil Bolognese or a chickpea and quinoa bowl are perfect examples of how pulses can elevate a dish.

7. Baking with Pulses: Pulses can even be used in baking! Chickpea flour is a gluten-free alternative that can be used in pancakes, cookies, and breads. Black beans can be blended into brownie batter for a fudgy, protein-rich dessert.

Embracing Pulses: A Step Toward a Healthier, Greener Diet

Incorporating pulses into your diet is a simple and delicious way to explore plant-based eating. Not only do they offer a host of health benefits, but they also contribute to a more sustainable food system. Whether you're making a complete transition to a plant-based diet or just looking to cut back on meat, pulses provide a versatile, nutritious, and environmentally friendly alternative to animal proteins.

By choosing pulses, you're not just nourishing your body—

you're also making a positive impact on the planet. So next time you plan your meals, consider adding these green proteins to your plate. Your health, and the environment, will thank you.

10

Gluten, Modified Grains, and the Dark Side of Commercial Cereals

ast but not least, I want to inform you about Gluten and hidden Sugars.

Many might have a problem with this, Or perhaps not even be aware of it. Gluten intolerance is quite common and under valued by doctors. Our favorite breakfast is overnight rolled oats with berries and almond milk. Or any milk of your choice. Give it a try!

Or bake your own bread with Emmer, Spelt or other non GMO grains. Like my Old Roman Spelt Bread!

Many of us reach for a box of cereal to start our day, believing it to be a quick and convenient breakfast option. However, what many don't realise is that these commercial cereals often contain ingredients that do more harm than good. From gluten and modified grains to excessive sugars, the contents of that innocent-looking box might be more of a "serial killer" than a healthy start to your day.

I make my own muesli with different organic nuts and coconut flakes , add them in my yogurt and top with berries.

Gluten and Modified Grains: What You Need to Know

Gluten, a protein found in wheat, barley, and rye, has become a hot topic in recent years. For those with celiac disease, gluten can cause serious health issues, but even for those without this condition, gluten from heavily modified grains can lead to digestive discomfort, inflammation, and other chronic health problems.

Over the decades, the grains used in most commercial foods have been genetically modified and processed to increase yields and profits. Unfortunately, this modification has come at a cost— these grains are often stripped of their nutrients and loaded with chemicals. The end result is a product that bears little resemblance to the wholesome, nutritious grains our ancestors consumed.

The Sugar Trap in Commercial Cereals

Perhaps even more alarming than the presence of gluten and modified grains is the sheer amount of sugar in commercial cereals. Many popular brands are loaded with sugars, artificial flavors, and preservatives—turning what should be a nutritious meal into a sugary, processed concoction that can spike your blood sugar levels and contribute to long-term health issues like obesity, diabetes, and heart disease.

A bowl of cereal may look harmless, but when you consider that some brands pack more sugar than a candy bar, it's clear that this is not the way to fuel your body for the day ahead. Eating these cereals regularly can set you on a path toward poor health, with little to no nutritional benefit.

The Better Way: Choose Whole Foods

Instead of reaching for that box of cereal, consider starting your day with whole, unprocessed foods. Oatmeal made from organic rolled oats, a smoothie packed with fruits, vegetables, and plant-based proteins, or even a simple slice of whole grain toast with avocado can offer the nutrients and energy your body truly needs.

By staying away from gluten-laden, sugar-filled commercial cereals, and choosing whole, organic foods instead, you can make a significant difference in your health. It's a simple change with profound effects—one that will help you start your day the right way.

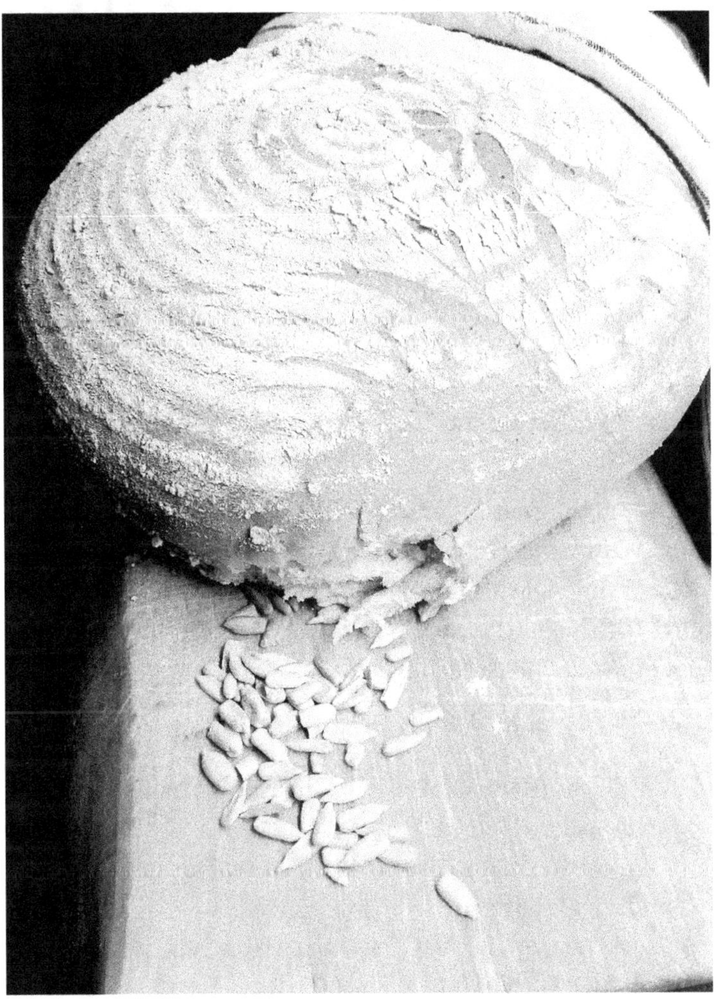

My home made Old Roman Spelt Bread

11

Organic Kitchen Pantry Shopping List

Building an organic kitchen starts with stocking up on wholesome, high-quality ingredients. Here's a shopping list to help you create a well-rounded pantry filled with pulses, grains, spices, and other essentials that support a nutritious, sustainable diet.

Pulses (Dried or Canned)

- Chickpeas (Garbanzo Beans): Versatile for hummus, stews, and salads.
- Lentils (Green, Red, Brown, Black): Great for soups, curries, and veggie burgers.
- Black Beans: Perfect for Mexican dishes, salads, and protein-rich dips.
- Kidney Beans: Ideal for chili, stews, and mixed bean salads.
- Pinto Beans: Common in refried beans, soups, and burritos.
- Navy Beans: Excellent for baked beans, soups, and stews.
- Split Peas (Green, Yellow): For hearty soups and purees.
- Mung Beans: Used in soups, salads, and Indian dals.
- Fava Beans: Great for spreads like fava bean hummus or in

Mediterranean dishes.
- Adzuki Beans: Common in Asian dishes and sweet bean pastes.

Whole Grains and Seeds

- Quinoa: High-protein grain for salads, bowls, and as a rice alternative.
- Brown Rice: Nutritious and filling, perfect for stir-fries, bowls, and sides.
- Oats: For breakfast, baking, and thickening smoothies.
- Barley: Excellent in soups, stews, and grain salads.
- Farro: A chewy, nutty grain for salads and pilafs.
- Chia Seeds: Rich in omega-3, ideal for puddings, smoothies, and baking.
- Flax seeds: Ground for smoothies, baking, and as an egg substitute.
- Hemp Seeds: For adding protein to smoothies, salads, and baking.

Nuts and Nut Butters

- Almonds: For snacking, baking, and making almond milk.
- Cashews: For creamy sauces, vegan cheeses, and snacks.
- Walnuts: Rich in omega-3s, great for baking, salads, and snacking.
- Peanut Butter: Organic, for spreads, sauces, and baking.
- Tahini: Sesame seed paste used in dressings, hummus, and sauces.

Oils and Fats

- Extra Virgin Olive Oil: For dressings, cooking, and drizzling.
- Coconut Oil: For cooking, baking, and as a dairy alternative.
- Avocado Oil: High heat cooking and salad dressings.
- Sesame Oil: For Asian-inspired dishes and dressings.
- Ghee (Clarified Butter): Organic, for high-heat cooking and traditional recipes.

Spices and Seasonings

- Turmeric: Anti-inflammatory, used in curries, stews, and golden milk.
- Cumin: Earthy spice for curries, soups, and spice blends.
- Coriander: Citrus-like flavor, used in spice blends, marinades, and curries.
- Paprika (Sweet, Smoked): Adds color and depth to stews, rubs, and sauces.
- Cinnamon: For baking, breakfast dishes, and savory stews.
- Ginger (Dried, Fresh): For adding warmth to dishes, teas, and baking.
- Garlic (Fresh, Powdered): A kitchen essential for almost any dish.
- Sea Salt: Unrefined, for seasoning and finishing dishes.
- Black Pepper: Freshly ground for seasoning everything from soups to salads.
- Nutritional Yeast: For a cheesy flavour in vegan dishes, soups, and sauces.
- Dried Herbs (Basil, Oregano, Thyme, Rosemary): Essential for flavouring a variety of dishes.

Pantry Staples

- Organic Canned Tomatoes: For sauces, soups, and stews.
- Tomato Paste: Concentrated flavor for sauces and stews.
- Vegetable Broth: For soups, stews, and cooking grains.
- Coconut Milk: For curries, soups, and creamy desserts.
- Apple Cider Vinegar: For dressings, marinades, and detox drinks.
- Soy Sauce or Tamari: For Asian dishes and savory seasoning.
- Maple Syrup or Honey: Natural sweeteners for baking, cooking, and dressings.

Fresh Produce (Store or Buy Locally)

- Garlic: A kitchen essential for seasoning and flavor.
- Onions (Yellow, Red, Shallots): For flavor bases in many dishes.
- Root Vegetables (Carrots, Potatoes, Sweet Potatoes): Long-lasting and versatile.
- Leafy Greens (Spinach, Kale, Swiss Chard): For salads, soups, and sides.
- Seasonal Vegetables: Based on what's fresh and available at farmers markets.

Finding Farmers Markets in the U.S.

Buying from farmers markets is a great way to support local agriculture, ensure the freshness of your produce, and reduce your environmental footprint. Here are some tips and resources for finding farmers markets across the U.S.:

1. USDA Farmers Market Directory: The U.S. Department of Agriculture maintains a comprehensive directory of farmers markets across the country. You can search by

location to find markets near you. Visit the directory at USDA Farmers Market Directory.

2. Local Harvest: This website connects consumers with local farmers, markets, and CSAs (Community Supported Agriculture). You can search for farmers markets, organic farms, and local food events by entering your zip code. Check out their directory at LocalHarvest.org.

3. Farmers Market Coalition: An organization dedicated to supporting farmers markets. Their website provides a wealth of resources, including a directory of markets and tips for shopping at farmers markets. Explore more at Farmers Market Coalition.

4. State and Local Resources: Many states have their own directories or websites dedicated to local farmers markets. For example, California's Certified Farmers Markets (CFM) or New York's GrowNYC Greenmarkets. A quick online search with your state name and "farmers market direc-tory" can help you find specific resources.

5. Apps and Social Media: Apps like Farmers Market Finder or Market Wagon can help you locate nearby markets. Additionally, following local farmers markets on social media can keep you updated on their offerings, hours, and special events.

By stocking your pantry with these essentials and seeking out fresh produce from farmers markets, you can create a kitchen that's ready to support a healthy, sustainable lifestyle. Whether you're cooking up a batch of hearty lentil soup, blending a chickpea-based dip, or crafting a quinoa salad, these ingredients will help you explore the vibrant world of plant-based and organic cooking. Plus, by shopping locally and seasonally, you're not only feeding your body with nutritious food but also supporting your community and the environment.

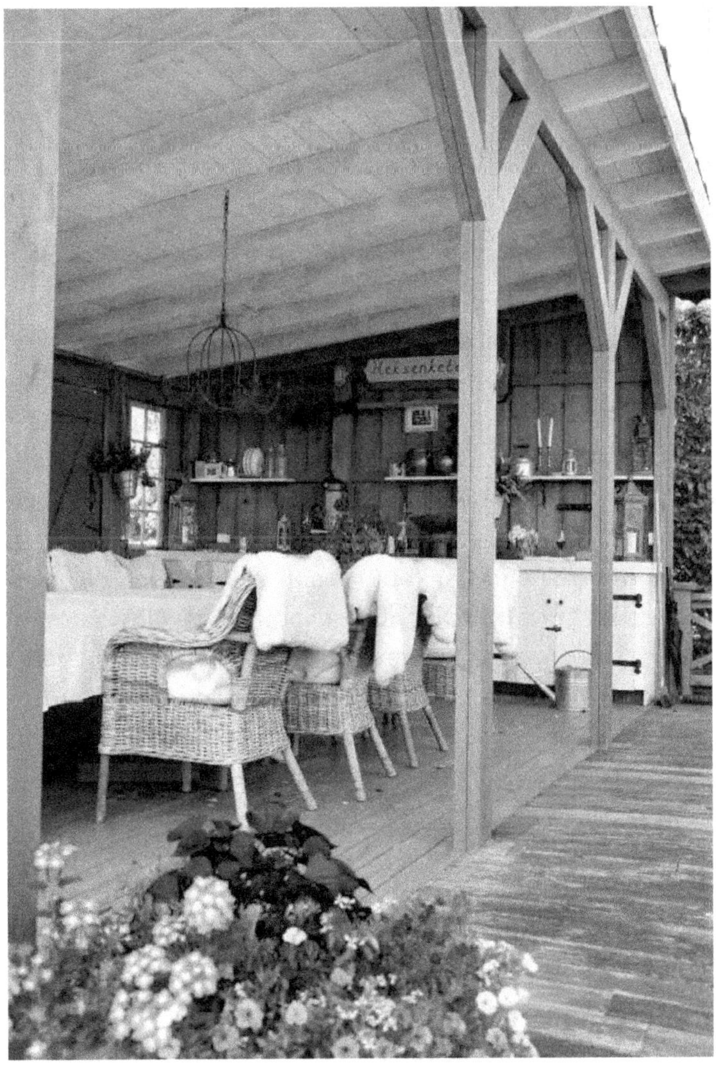

12

Conclusion

A <u>Call to Conscious Consumption</u>

Choosing your greens , meat and fish and grains wisely is about more than just what's on your plate—it's about making informed decisions that benefit your health, the environment, and the wider community. By opting for organic, local, and whole foods, you not only reduce your exposure to harmful chemicals but also support sustainable farming practices that nurture the planet. Every time you choose organic or buy from a local farmer, you're making a statement: you care about what you eat, where it comes from, and how it's grown. In doing so, you're not just feeding your body—you're nourishing your soul and supporting a healthier world.

Remember, the choices we make today in the supermarket or in the restaurant will shape the world we live in tomorrow.

If you are living in the city or travelling the world as a digital nomad, or just living in a sleepy small town or even own your own island in the tropics, we all need real good food, to stay healthy.

Our organic sheep farm and vegetable garden are more than just sources of food—they're a way of life, a source of joy, and a connection to the natural world. By gardening with the moon, sowing in the spring with high-quality seeds from The Bolster, and embracing the entire growing season, we find purpose and fulfilment in every step of the journey.

As we sit down to a meal made from the fruits of our labour, we're reminded that this is what life is all about—working with our hands, nurturing the earth, and enjoying the simple, profound pleasures of a life well lived.

Learn More Tips:

Food Supplements are useful to support your body to keep detoxing. Find a Natural Holistic Doctor to guide you, or try MINDVALLEY App course 'the Ultimate Guide to Supplements.

Stay informed about Food, my favourite Podcast is FOOD TALK, of course there is more to discover.

Celebrate Real Food!

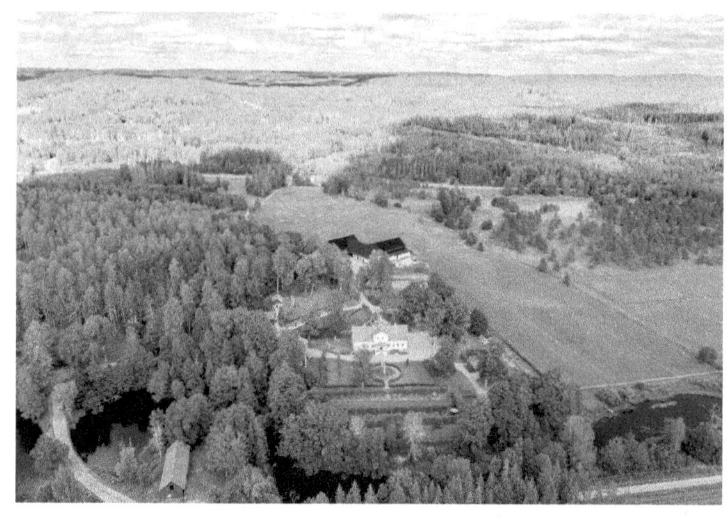

Epilogue

To plant an organic garden is to believe in the future

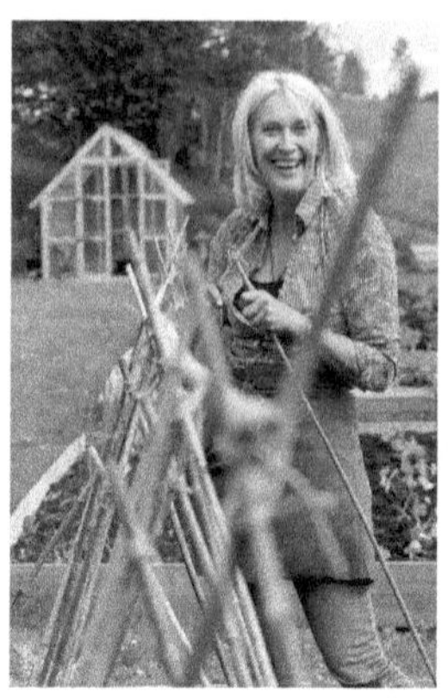

About the Author

Karin Kalteren Busink is a passionate advocate for real food and better health, living on an organic farm in the serene landscapes of Sweden with her husband and two beloved dogs. With a rich background in the food supplement industry and as a nutritionist, Karin has dedicated her life to exploring the profound connection between nutrition and well-being. Her love for organic farming and commitment to supporting local farmers and farmers' markets is at the heart of her work. Karin believes in the power of natural, wholesome foods to nourish both body and soul. Through her writings, she shares her insights on the importance of sustainable agriculture and the benefits of choosing organic, locally-sourced produce. Whether she's tending to her farm, sharing her knowledge on nutrition, or writing to inspire others, Karin's mission remains clear: to help people embrace healthier lifestyles through the simple yet powerful choices they make every day.

9 7 9 8 3 3 3 5 8 5 3 1 1 8